A SINGLE STEP

How to look after your health through your feet.

Kate McEwan

A SINGLE STEP
How to look after your health through your feet.
First edition – published in September 2016
Copyright © 2016 Kate McEwan
The right of Kate McEwan to be identified as the author of this work has been asserted by her in accordance with the Copyright Designs and Patents Act 1988.
All rights reserved. No part of this book may be reproduced in any material form (including photocopying or storing in any medium by electronic means and whether or not transiently or incidentally to some other use of this publication) without the written permission of the copyright holder except in accordance with the provisions of the Copyright, Design and Patents Act 1988. Applications for the Copyright holder's written permission to reproduce any part of this publication should be addressed to the author.
The information provided in this book should not be treated as a substitute for professional medical advice; always consult a medical practitioner. Any use of information in this book is at the readers' discretion and risk. Neither the author nor the publisher can be held responsible for any loss, claim or damage arising out of the use, or misuse, of the suggestions made, the failure to take medical advice or for any material on third party websites.
A CIP catalogue record for this book is available from the British Library.
ISBN : 978-0-9957635-0-0

To my father, who taught me to never give up, and to David, who has taught me everything I know about joy.

Contents

Acknowledgements 7
Introduction   9

Part One: Health   11

An Act of Love 13
How Will Looking After Your Feet Help Your General Health? 15
Managing Lifestyle Changes So They Stick 19
The Importance of Rest   21
The Importance of Good Hydration   25
Why You Should Drink Lemon Water 27
Diet and Exercise 31

Part Two: Reflexology 33

Different Types of Medicine: Western, Complementary and Holistic   35
The Emotional Aspects of Reflexology 39
My Reflexology Heroes   41
Improve Fertility Naturally 43
Pregnancy and Reflexology 47
Reflexology and Menopause   51

Manage Anxiety Naturally Using Reflexology 55
Reflexology and Back Pain 59
Reflexology and IBS 61
Migraine – A Case Study 63

Part Three: Foot Healthcare 67

What should you do if you have a pain in your foot? 69
Swimming Pools and Changing Rooms 71
Runner's Foot Problems 73
High Heels 77
Natural treatment for a verruca 81
Hard Skin and Callus 85
Home-made Foot Scrub Recipe 89
How to deal with corns 91
Fungal Nail Infections 95
Foot Care for Diabetics 97

Final Word 99

Acknowledgements

I have a lot of people to thank for their help during this process. Firstly my family for their continued love and support throughout the writing of this book.

My soul family, especially Jess Pitman, who never doubts me, always supports me and catches me when I stumble.

Hannah Chambers and Bernard Pink for training me so comprehensively in the fields of Reflexology and Foot Healthcare, and for encouraging my natural inclination to ethical practice.

Neil Wilkins, for challenging me to write this during our strategy sessions, and your enduring faith in my ability to do it.

Inge Dowden, for being my biggest cheerleader, and holding me accountable so I kept on pushing forward.

Mark Gautieri, for the beautiful cover design which totally reflects the spirit and feeling of the book.

Ann Hobbs, Amy Morse, Helen Blenkinsop, and Marie J Taylor for all the practical advice which ensured this book was published, and not relegated to a dusty cupboard in the cloud.

Introduction

With advances in health over the last 100 years the Western population is living longer. This has brought with it consequences, including many illnesses directly related to old age, but also many illnesses which, while not age related, have a massive effect on the quality of life for the elderly.

I grew up in a household where my mother's health was a constant topic of conversation. If it wasn't her back, it was a migraine, and she was constantly taking one pill or another. Her dependence on western medicine was total and yet she never got any better. She was an incredibly hard working woman who averaged 50 to 60 hours a week, until eventually she stopped work due to ill-health, and never returned to work. She was diagnosed with ME and then struggled with that until her death.

My father on the face of it was far healthier. He never had colds or needed to take time off work. He too worked long hours, until the 80s recession hit. However, although he seemed healthy, his diet was very high in red meat and dairy products, and he was a chain smoker.

He was diagnosed with lung cancer at age 52 and died two years later.

He died when I was 23, and one year later I stopped smoking and embarked on a total change of lifestyle. I had seen for myself that what I had grown up with, didn't work. Western medicine hadn't been able to keep my father alive. On some level I decided that I didn't want to die young, but that also left a huge question. It is easy to say you don't want to die young. People want to live to see their grandchildren. But how did I want to live?

It was obvious to me that I didn't want to decline gradually into old age, dragging along a huge list of ailments. I wanted to be the 80 year old in the swimming pool, doing my hour every morning. For me there was no point in living a long time if I couldn't live well!

Part One: Health

"A journey of a thousand miles begins with a single step."
Confucius

An Act of Love

For most people feet are the least desirable part of the body. Often people have very negative feelings towards them. Some people are even more extreme, claiming to hate their own feet. "I can't stand feet", "I can't bear anyone touching my feet", are phrases I hear frequently when talking about what I do. I'm asked, "How can you bear to touch peoples feet every day?" When describing feet, the language is often negative. They are fat, smelly or ugly.

To me this is very sad. Firstly, feet need looking after, however negatively people feel about them. Without feet we would not be able to move around, and if we have anything painful on our feet, we become deeply aware of them. Imagine how it feels, if every step we take causes pain? Perhaps you don't have to.

More than this though, our feet are an essential part of our body. I think it is truly a tragedy to loathe a part of yourself. To have deeply negative feelings towards such an essential part of ourselves is wrong. If we can't love and accept ourselves, how can we love and accept others?

We need to view any form of self-care as an act of love, and our feet perhaps more than most parts of the body deserve that. What is the point of spending hundreds of pounds on our outward appearance if our feet are crying out for attention? If we care about ourselves we need to care about our whole selves, and not just the parts which show.

How Will Looking After Your Feet Help Your General Health?

This book came about largely out of my own desire to stay well. I believe that we should be proactive in our approach to health, not just reacting when things go wrong. Just as rest, diet and exercise are crucial to this, so I believe, is using a therapy such as Reflexology. It is important to deal with health problems as they arise. Issues which start off as a slight inconvenience can turn into a huge problem if neglected.

One of the reasons it is important to use Reflexology to stay healthy, is because a Reflexologist can pick up issues on the feet before the person is even aware that there is a problem. If a person complains of having a sore throat, the Reflexologist will not only work on the throat, but also on the immune system to start working against any possible infection, and on the adrenal glands to work against any inflammation.

Using Reflexology as a therapy to stay well

can work in many different ways. Reflexologists work on the immune system to help the body's ability to fight disease. As I mentioned above, a treatment at the right time can work on minor symptoms to prevent them getting worse. It can also work to speed up the healing process of an illness that has fully developed.

We work on the digestive system to ensure that nutrients and waste are processed well by the body. Ensuring the body eliminates waste regularly and efficiently can have a preventative effect. People who have trouble moving their bowels can end up with more serious problems such as diverticulitis. Because Reflexology encourages the body to eliminate, regular treatment can help regularise bowel movements.

This is just one example of how Reflexology through the feet can help individuals maintain a state of good health. I will explore a few areas in more detail later in this book. For now I would like to briefly explore more obvious ways in which looking after your feet can help your health.

In my clinical experience as a Foot Health

Practitioner I tend to see a lot of people with painful feet. Because we tend to be using our feet most of the time, any kind of pain is very debilitating. Any kind of pain in the foot immediately affects the way we walk. It is natural to try and modify our gait to minimise pain, but this can only lead to change in posture. Any change in posture can lead to more serious issues in the skeletal system. Anything which causes us to change the way we walk can put parts of the skeletal system out of alignment which can lead to pain and other problems.

For this reason it is essential that if you have a painful problem on your foot you pay attention and seek treatment. Looking after your feet when they need it can prevent other problems developing. I have gone into more detail in the following chapters about specific problems which can develop on the feet. I will talk about what causes them, and what we can do ourselves to prevent and treat them ourselves.

"We are what we repeatedly do. Excellence, then, is not an act, but a habit." Aristotle

Managing Lifestyle Changes So They Stick

Most attempts at lifestyle changes flounder because they are too large and overwhelming. If your aim was to improve your diet, why not start with just one change, and make it positive. Introduce one new thing into your routine, like drinking more water, or eating more fruit, and try to keep that up for three weeks. By the end of three weeks it will have become a habit, and then you can try introducing another positive change.

Another reason efforts to improve lifestyle fall by the wayside, is because they are framed in a negative way. People talk about giving up, which creates a feeling of deprivation around their goal. So instead of giving up smoking, why not just stop smoking?

 Any lifestyle change around food, which focuses on not being able to have certain things, as most diets do, may become unsustainable in the long term. Try introducing more fruit, vegetables and legumes into your diet. If you crowd your meals with nutrient rich healthy food, you will have less room in your stomach for rubbish.

Do your good intentions cost money? Gym memberships can be really expensive and unless you are someone who loves the gym and already has a habit of going two or three times a week, you may end up not getting your money's worth. If you want to go to a gym as part of your exercise routine, but aren't sure about how committed you can be, most local leisure centres have a gym where you can pay as you go, just as you can with their swimming pools.

Why not try something completely free? If you drive to work every day, why not leave earlier and park a mile from your office, giving you a brisk walk before and after work. Walking before work will wake you up, and walking afterwards will help you process any stress and frustrations which built up in the day.

So if you have let your good intentions slip, don't beat yourself up. Just make one small change!

The Importance of Rest

Rest is one of the most undervalued aspects of our lives, and yet it is one of the most important. Without proper rest we slowly become run down, our immune system weakens, we become more prone to illness, and slowly but surely exhaustion can set in.

The need for rest is fundamental but it runs counter to the prevailing narrative of our time. We must be constantly active and busy. We must not waste time. We must be strivers not skivers!

I frequently meet people in my practice who make no connection with the fact that their health problems may be due to a lack of down time and rest. It is obvious really, that headaches towards the end of the day may be due to fatigue, but what if the consequences are more serious.

A good example of this is fertility. Most people acknowledge that stress can affect fertility but if you regard your lifestyle as normal, and you are not aware of the amount of stress you are under, it is possible to be limiting your chances of conceiving children.

Here is an example of how this might happen: Imagine this scenario. A couple in their late 30s are trying to have their first baby. They both work 40 + hours a week in their high powered, extremely stressful jobs.

This impacts their ability to lead a healthy lifestyle, because after work and the gym they may not always have the energy to cook healthy meals. They continue to exercise by heading to the gym before work, but while this has some positive benefits, it also leads to their levels of depletion.

They are trying to conceive, but her fertility levels are starting to drop due to her age. His fertility might be compromised for any number of reasons (smoking, high caffeine or alcohol intake, the bout of flu he had last month.) They try to conceive for a year without success, during which stress levels rise, doubts and insecurities come in to play, and they finally seek medical help.

There begins a round of tests which may or may not find anything medically wrong. If it doesn't, they are back to square one, and will be offered a series of fertility interventions, which will only add to the stress levels of the couple. They are now experiencing one of the most stressful times of their lives.

When you are living in a situation it can be hard to look at it objectively and recognise all the things that are affecting you. In Part Two I explore in more detail some ways of improving fertility naturally.

There are many other situations where stress and lack of rest can be affecting health, which is why it is so important to take time for ourselves.

"Ah! There is nothing like staying at home, for real comfort."
Jane Austen

The Importance of Good Hydration

It is obvious to a Reflexologist when someone is dehydrated. Their feet can have a dry, leathery feel. If you are someone who suffers from dry, hard skin on your feet, one thing you should certainly review is how much water you drink.

There is a lot of conflicting advice on how much water we should drink. General guidelines say 2 litres a day, but if you participate in a high energy sport, that just won't be enough. Common sense is important here.

Being well hydrated is important because it supports the kidneys in the work they do removing impurities from the blood. Drinking too much water on the other hand, can overload the kidneys, so it is important not to go overboard.

Some people argue that the two litres should be made up of just water, while others argue that it can include any liquid. There is room for common sense here too. If we are working to support the kidney, then our aim is not to add to the burden. So I recommend including fluids like water, lemon water and herbal teas, but not including tea, coffee, alcohol or sugary drinks.

When you drink is important too. I believe it is a good idea to drink a large glass of water in the morning to help flush out the accumulation of toxins from the night before. I like to follow that with a cup of hot lemon water to continue the detoxifying process and stimulate the organs.

So how do you know if you are becoming dehydrated? Well thirst is an excellent sign, but it means that you are already dehydrated. Also be aware of the colour and smell of your urine. It should be pale and odourless. If it is a deep yellow, or even a brown colour with a strong smell you need to drink some water!

Why You Should Drink Lemon Water!

One thing my clients know well, is that I have a slight obsession with lemon water. I always have a bag of lemons in the fridge, and I wouldn't start the day without my mug of hot lemon water.

While hydration levels have an effect on the health of the whole body, they also have an effect on the condition of the feet, so it is essential to make sure you are getting enough fluids.

When I take a client's case history before working with them, we always talk about how much water they drink, and as most of them report a struggle with drinking enough water, I always recommend lemon water.

I've put together a short list of reasons why you should drink lemon water, some are very practical, and others are more for health reasons.

- Drinking lemon water is a good way to help you increase your water consumption. If you don't drink much water because you like hot drinks, then a quarter segment of lemon in a mug of hot water should solve that.

- If you only like drinks with flavour, then you can't find anything which tastes nicer than fresh sharp lemon.

- Dehydration can cause headaches and fatigue, which is one of the most important reasons why you should drink lemon water.

- A mug of hot lemon water is a great way to start your day. Lemons contain negatively charged ions which help increase energy naturally as they enter the digestive tract.

- Lemon water boosts your vitamin C intake. Lemons are a rich source of vitamin C, and a few cups a day, will significantly increase your levels. Vitamin C has a vital role in preventing cell damage, and in supporting your immune system, which can help prevent you from becoming ill.

- Lemon water is very good for digestion. It

helps the body to process food more slowly, which helps to prevent bloating. It stimulates the liver, which helps remove toxins.

• Because it contains pectin, which helps you feel full, drinking lemon water can help with weight loss over time.

• It tastes delicious. If you only need one reason why you should drink lemon water, then this should be it!

I hope by now you are inspired to start your new habit of drinking lemon water every day. There are plenty of variations on how you can drink it, but my method is very simple. I quarter a lemon, and squeeze it into a mug, and drop the squeezed quarter in as well. Then, just top with boiling water. The beauty of this method, is that it tastes good hot and cold, so it really doesn't make any difference if you forget about it for a while.

"Pure water is the world's first and foremost medicine."
Slovak Proverb

Diet and Exercise

I am neither a qualified nutritional therapist nor a fitness instructor, so I am not going to go into great detail about diet and exercise. Rather I will just include a brief summary of a few principles to follow.

The concept of eating the rainbow (not Skittles!) is one I very much subscribe to. I believe to be healthy everyone should be eating a diet rich in all kinds of fresh fruit and vegetables. I also believe that eating protein derived from plant sources such as beans and pulses is much more beneficial for health than animal protein. For an easily accessible summary of the scientific support for this approach, I recommend watching the film Forks over Knives.

Regular exercise is generally regarded as one of the pillars of a healthy lifestyle, but I believe it is important to carefully choose how you exercise. I believe in a balance of aerobic exercise such as swimming, combined with yoga or Pilates, and some form of weight bearing exercise such as resistance training. I strongly believe that extreme sporting challenges should be undertaken infrequently, and forms of exercise such as running should be enjoyed moderately.

"I have to exercise in the morning before my brain figures out what I'm doing."
Marsha Doble

Part Two: Reflexology

"Forget not that the earth delights to feel your bare feet and the winds long to play with your hair."
Khalil Gibran

Different Types of Medicine: Western, Complementary and Holistic

Although the terms are used interchangeably, there is a very important difference between the idea of alternative medicine and complementary medicine. Using the term alternative medicine, gives the impression from the person using it (hopefully unintentionally) that they see the therapy as a complete alternative to western medicine.

I say, "hopefully unintentionally" because I firmly believe that no therapy should be used as a complete alternative to western medicine, and that is why I use the term complementary. A complementary practitioner should work alongside the medical profession, collaborating where possible, with the common goal of helping the client return to good health.

Western medicine has made massive strides in our knowledge of the pathology (the process) of disease, and crucially it has hugely increased the health, wellbeing and longevity of the general population. Access to free healthcare and dental care has undoubtedly meant that many people who would otherwise have succumbed to disease and death, have lived. Where it fails, in my opinion, is that Western doctors tend to look no further than the symptom they are presented with. This means in practise, that if you go to see a Doctor about headaches, they will generally treat the symptom by giving you painkillers, but not enquire into what is causing the headaches.

When you see a complementary therapy practitioner they should begin by taking a complete health history, and at every subsequent visit they will review your symptoms since the last treatment. Through this process they would be able to see patterns, and consequently raise questions about what might be leading to the headaches. Back pain causing you to hunch? Constant staring at a screen for work? Chronic constipation? Headaches linked to the menstrual cycle?

The wonderful thing about a therapy like Reflexology though, is that it is holistic. During every treatment the therapist should work on every part of your body. This means that even if no one knows what is causing your symptoms, they may resolve through treatment, because if the therapist is working on every part of your body, they will most likely work on the area at the root of the problem. This is why I firmly believe in treatments with a holistic approach, and it is why I never give shortened treatments as part of a long term approach.

I trained as a Reflexologist 13 years ago in a private school in mid Wales with an exceptional teacher, Hannah Chambers.
I had decided to start a career in holistic healthcare because I wanted to change my life into one with focus and passion. Although I came to the therapy with a great deal of interest I could never have dreamed how fascinating and incredible it could be.

One of the things which has always frustrated me in my career as a Reflexologist is how many people have a perception of it (if they have heard of it at all) as simply a relaxing therapy. Unless people have direct experience, very little is known in the wider community about its therapeutic value; and yet on a daily basis I meet people who walk away feeling better as a result of it. People are very often happy to try acupuncture as a treatment, where they would not even consider Reflexology.

Reflexology and Acupuncture are both energy medicines, which means that they both follow the principle that energy runs though the body along channels or meridians, and that blockages in the flow of that energy can lead to problems in the health of the body. And in both therapies, practitioners intervene at points of the body to help release those blockages and allow the energy to flow freely again. Reflexology is best known for using reflexes on the feet to do this, but you will hear of practitioners using points on the hands, ears and other places.

For my money, Reflexology is most effective when used on the feet for two main reasons: firstly the Reflexes on the feet offer a complete map of the body, and so it is possible to do a completely holistic treatment on the feet. Secondly, Foot Reflexology is incredibly pleasant and relaxing, which adds another level to the treatment. It just feels really good!

The Emotional Aspects of Reflexology

Reflexology is a very physical therapy. We work on the body, primarily on the feet, although some therapists use reflexes on the hands and ears, among other areas, as well.

Most people who are familiar with Reflexology know that we work certain specific reflexes to effect change in other areas of the body. This is the most obvious aspect of Reflexology, but it is not the only way in which the therapy works.

As already discussed, Reflexology is an energy medicine, and as such, works on the energy running through the body to bring about optimum health and well-being. These subtle energy systems are very complex, and the way a therapist works can have a profound effect on the nature of the treatment. In my practise I use a gentle but focused touch specifically to work on the subtle energy systems.

Reflexology works well on a mechanical level to bring about immediate relief for presenting symptoms, but the magic really begins to happen when a therapist uses their many layers of knowledge to work the physical aspects of the body, intuitively accessing the subtle energy systems. The change and healing can be deep and profound. Clients may find themselves experiencing memories from long ago, and connecting those memories with physical problems they are currently experiencing. They can make connections with emotional traumas which are still affecting decisions in their day to day lives.

Different areas of the body have different emotional significance and a therapist who works on a deeper level will have a knowledge of the emotional aspects of the areas they are working on. For example the lungs relate strongly to the desire for life, and so the occurrence of respiratory disorders can indicate an issue around the individual's right to draw breath. The respiratory system is also an area where grief is held in the body. It is not uncommon for a person having their first Reflexology treatment to become very emotional when the lungs are being worked upon.

My Reflexology Heroes

Did you know Reflexology was rediscovered in the west by a surgeon, Dr William Fitzgerald?

He was born in 1872 in the United States, and became a leading ear, nose and throat surgeon, working in Boston, London and Vienna.

He developed the concept of Zone Therapy while he was senior nose and throat surgeon in Connecticut.

He observed while working that if he applied pressure over certain points of the toes, feet and other parts of the body, it caused a type of anaesthesia in a limited area. This enabled him to perform minor operations on the nose and throat without using cocaine and other local analgesics.

He went on to teach this technique to Dr Joseph Shelby-Riley and his wife Elizabeth who used this method in their practise for many years.

Riley's assistant, Eunice Ingham (1879 – 1974) advanced Reflexology dramatically when she separated the reflexes on the feet from Zone Therapy in general.

Working as a physiotherapist with Dr Shelby-Riley, she had the opportunity to check and recheck each reflex point on hundreds of patients. She felt that the feet should be special targets for therapy because of their highly sensitive nature, and she eventually evolved on the feet themselves a "map" of the entire body.

Her contribution is acknowledged to be so great that she is known as the mother of Reflexology, and is credited with being the founder of foot Reflexology. Most Reflexology charts are based on her work.

Improve Fertility Naturally

Fertility problems, and the process of undergoing conventional fertility treatment, are now widely acknowledged to be one of the most stressful experiences that an individual can experience. Small wonder then, that so many people look for ways to improve fertility naturally.

I suggest to my clients that they should picture how they imagine their future life with their new baby, and as far as is possible, try to make their life now match that. An essential part of overcoming fertility issues is looking at a couples' lifestyle and expectations.

People have an expectation that they can work hard until their 40's to get their lives to a certain point, and then have children when they want. Unfortunately, a woman's ability to conceive starts to drop dramatically in her late 30s, so one factor to consider if a person wants to improve fertility naturally, is making positive lifestyle changes in order to optimise health.

There are many small changes that women

and men can make to improve fertility naturally and these are part of a process of making positive lifestyle changes. Smoking, alcohol and caffeine all have a negative effect on a person's fertility, and so addressing these habits should be the first place to start.

Before couples even think about consulting a doctor, they should be looking at these factors. A study by Klonoff-Cohen et al (2002) found that consumption of alcohol and caffeine was a risk factor for not achieving a live birth (either by not becoming pregnant or due to miscarriage.)

Fertility and stress are often linked, but there is no conclusive scientific evidence that stress has an adverse effect on fertility. However stress can have an effect on the endocrine system and the appropriate production of hormones, and so if a couple are trying to improve fertility naturally, both partners should be evaluating how much stress there is in their lives and take steps to reduce it.

Certain factors such as: poor sperm quality or mobility, can make a huge difference to a couple's ability to conceive, and so a good understanding of how this is positively and negatively affected is important to improve fertility naturally. It takes about 3 months for new sperm to fully mature, which means that something like a bad virus with a fever can kill sperm and reduce fertility dramatically for 3 months. Additionally, as alcohol and caffeine consumption have an effect on sperm production, this three month life cycle should be considered, while waiting for sperm quality to improve.

A regular menstrual cycle is also critical in conception. If a woman's cycle is extremely irregular, she will not be ovulating, but even small variations in the length of a cycle can have significant impact on how often a woman ovulates.

Some of the greatest success I have had in my clinic have been with women in this position. They have been struggling to get pregnant, but no one has really talked about how vital having a regular menstrual cycle is. A menstrual cycle with less than 12 days between ovulation and menstruation can be problematic because the mucous membrane in the uterus needs time to prepare for the fertilized egg. We work together to reduce their stress and bring their endocrine system back into balance, so that they can have the best chance of ovulating. A client of mine, Sarah, fell pregnant within weeks of her cycle becoming regular.

Because Reflexology is so relaxing it naturally helps individuals in times of stress. For couples undergoing different types of fertility treatment, anything that reduces their stress can help improve the likely success of the treatment.

Below is a website address for further information on the effects of caffeine, alcohol and smoking on fertility:

http://yourfertility.org.au/Effects-of-caffeine-alcohol-and-smoking-on-fertility.pdf

Pregnancy and Reflexology

Pregnancy is undoubtedly one of the most wonderful experiences a woman can have, but the huge demands it places on the body can lead to quite a number of problems. Morning sickness, back pain, constipation and fatigue are commonly associated with the stages of pregnancy but they don't have to be just accepted. These symptoms can be managed and reduced with Reflexology.

Reflexology is a fantastic way to prepare a woman's body for labour, and can be effectively used during labour as well. Because Reflexology helps women during pregnancy to relax and connect with the process, it can have a very positive influence on the length and progress of labour.

Morning sickness is one of the most common experiences of pregnancy and it can become extremely severe. It is actually a really positive sign of a healthy pregnancy, but that may not be of much comfort when going through it. It is caused by the surges in progesterone in the early stages of pregnancy as the body prepares the uterus for expansion.

Fatigue is a common symptom of pregnancy which occurs particularly during the first trimester, but can affect women throughout the entire pregnancy. The best advice is to rest as much as possible, but using Reflexology can help to boost energy levels and reduce the impact of fatigue.

Back pain begins to be a factor towards the later stages of pregnancy, although it can affect women earlier. Reflexology works on the skeleton to relax and support it, and to release any tension or pain. I found this aspect extremely useful during my pregnancy, as I had a huge baby bump and had quite severe back pain at times.

Constipation is a common complaint in pregnancy because the foetus has grown to such a size that it is pushing into the organs surrounding it. Even women who don't have problems with constipation can experience some difficulties at this point. Again Reflexology works to help elimination, and ensure the nerve supply to the colon is working well. Women who have Reflexology from the start of their pregnancy often find they don't have any problems with constipation, but for women who do, even just one or two treatments can be enough to resolve them.

It is good to have weekly Reflexology treatments during pregnancy, to help ensure you are in the best possible health. Even if, for whatever reason you can't have weekly treatments, seeing a Reflexologist a few times during your pregnancy will be beneficial.

Lotus Tips:

The three most important things to concentrate on during pregnancy are:

- **Rest**
- **Healthy diet**
- **Gentle exercise**

"The best and most beautiful things in the world cannot be seen or even touched — they must be felt with the heart."
Helen Keller

Reflexology and Menopause

Menopause is an important subject for a Reflexologist because almost all women will experience some symptoms.

Menopause is often regarded with dread, and as something to be avoided, (and/or medicated), but in my view it is a transition into a new stage of life.

Symptoms can vary - woman to woman - from a gradual decrease in periods, to an abrupt ending of them. The most common symptoms are hot flushes, dizziness and mood changes, and for some women these can be so severe as to be really debilitating, and the symptoms can go on for years.

Menopause is officially diagnosed when a woman has not menstruated for a full year, and the period before that is known as the perimenopause. During perimenopause, ovulation becomes less regular, oestrogen levels decrease and progesterone levels fluctuate.

The good news for women going through this transition, is that Reflexology can be beneficial to a woman at this time. Reflexology as a therapy is excellent at helping to balance hormone levels in the body, which in turn will help manage the symptoms of menopause. A skilled Reflexologist will work the endocrine system thoroughly, as part of a holistic treatment.

You might wonder why it is important to explore treatments such as Reflexology as a way of helping manage the symptoms of menopause. After all, most women are offered HRT by their GP's as symptoms start to appear. More and more scientific studies are showing a link between the use of HRT in menopause, and the development of breast cancer, so more women are looking for natural ways to manage without HRT, and Reflexology is one of those ways.

My advice to woman who are experiencing perimenopause or menopausal symptoms is to prioritise self-care. Listen to your body's rhythms, and obey your need for rest. Nourish yourself with good food. Take as much exercise as you can manage, and forgive yourself if the symptoms are so severe one day that you just can't manage it. The combination of a healthy lifestyle (a really good diet and exercise), rest and Reflexology is often enough to help women manage their symptoms without needing to seek extra medical support.

Lotus Tips

If you are experiencing menopausal symptoms, above all be kind to yourself.

- **Get plenty of rest**
- **Drink plenty of water**
- **Eat plenty of fruit and vegetables**
- **Exercise regularly**

"Keep your eyes on the stars, and your feet on the ground."
Theodore Roosevelt

Manage Anxiety Naturally Using Reflexology

Anxiety is something I often see in my clinic. People come to me with a variety of symptoms such as: insomnia, IBS, persistent headaches and exhaustion, and frequently anxiety is the common theme underpinning everything.

We are not brought up to be able to identify anxiety. Very often we are not taught to examine our emotions and look at the factors leading up to them. It is very rare that anyone even points out that the hectic pace of life and many demands on our time are not quite right and may be beyond our ability to cope with. Clients come to me with a few symptoms and describe juggling all sorts of demands and stresses, but do not identify that this all might be too much and they may be overloaded.

Actually it doesn't matter. The wonderful thing about Reflexology is that you don't need a diagnosis to be able to work well with complicated health problems. Because Reflexologists work holistically, a good practitioner will work on every area of the body.

Reflexology works to manage anxiety naturally in a number of ways. The first part of this process is time. By committing an hour to visit a Reflexologist an individual is sending a powerful message to their body, that they value it enough to prioritise self-care. For some people the hour in the Reflexologists chair is the only hour of true relaxation they have, and it is precious.

The second way Reflexology works to manage anxiety naturally is by encouraging people to review their lifestyle. During the initial consultation a thorough health history will be taken, which will cover the habits of day to day life and quickly flag up if someone is doing something like drinking too much caffeine, which could be aggravating their symptoms.

During treatments with my clients, I try to create a space where they can understand how different factors are affecting their lives, and allow them to acknowledge that they may have been more overwhelmed than they realise. It is very easy to ignore the fact that you are overworked, "because that's just the way it has to be." If a person can identify that, they then have the power to make changes to bring themselves back into balance.

The third way in which Reflexology helps people to manage anxiety naturally is directly through the treatment. All treatments begin with a warm up of the feet, and then move on to the relaxation reflexes. There are areas in the body which particularly hold tension, and if these are relaxed, the whole body can let go. Following this there are specific reflexes on the feet which we can work on to help calm the body and reduce anxiety. The principle reflex is the adrenal glands on each foot. The adrenal gland governs the secretion of adrenaline in stressful situations, so working this reflex is essential during every treatment.

Reflexology is an excellent way to manage anxiety naturally, both in a crisis situation and as a long term strategy. Rather as people service their cars regularly, I believe people benefit from having regular Reflexology sessions. Having a treatment once a month, helps a healthy individual support their body, and stay in balance.

When you arise in the morning, think of what a precious privilege it is to be alive - to breathe, to think, to enjoy, to love.
Marcus Aurelius

Reflexology and Back Pain

Anyone reading this who has suffered from back pain will know what a debilitating problem it is. Back pain can range from mild to severe, but it is always life-limiting and always causes a disruption in our day to day lives.

According to a study published by Nuffield Health in 2015, up to 6 million people in the UK are living with undiagnosed back pain, and in 2013 it was the cause of more than 15 million sick days. You can find the study here:

http://www.nuffieldhealth.com/article/six-million-britons-living-with-undiagnosed-back-pain

The usual treatment from a GP begins with painkillers, and then depending on the severity of the problem can move into physiotherapy, and surgical intervention. But as anyone who has experienced this knows, these treatments can be limited in their effectiveness, and can lead to people just "living with it."

The skeleton is a complex mechanism, with the spine providing the stability and strength for the movement of the limbs. Any slight imbalance can cause postural changes which ultimately lead to discomfort or pain in another area of the skeleton.

There is no quick fix as far as back pain is concerned, and in my opinion, individuals who are recovering from a back injury should be looking at a combination of exercise and therapy to promote long-term recovery.

A Reflexologist will work on the whole of the skeletal system, firstly to relieve painful symptoms, but also to work on areas which may be aggravating the problem. Direct pressure on the skeletal reflexes will help relieve pain, while working on the adrenal glands will relieve any inflammation which will also result in pain relief. A combination of this kind of treatment coupled with gentle exercises can help resolve many back problems quite quickly.

Reflexology and IBS

It is never a surprise to me when I am taking a client's health history, if they mention they suffer from Irritable Bowel Syndrome, or IBS. It is an extremely common condition but it can be very unpleasant. It is a condition that responds really well to treatment with Reflexology.

Symptoms of IBS include diarrhoea and / or constipation, stomach cramps and bloating. The symptoms can be severe and extremely painful. Some people only experience symptoms after eating certain foods, and find that simply cutting out those foods is enough to stop the symptoms.

Other people find that they have symptoms whatever they eat. In these situations it is common to find that stress is an underlying factor. Reflexology really comes into its own here, and as a therapist it is in these situations that I have seen the most dramatic results. Reflexology is so intensely relaxing, that it often only takes a couple of treatments to see the symptoms improve. If an individual has a very stressful lifestyle then it can be beneficial to continue having monthly treatments, to prevent symptoms again.

As I have mentioned earlier in the book, Reflexology is effective in these cases because it is a holistic treatment. A good Reflexologist will treat the whole system. So, not only the digestive system will be worked, but also the reflexes governing the nerve supply to the digestive organs, and reflexes associated with the stress response, the adrenal glands. Treating only the symptoms would do nothing for the underlying causes, and so would not be as effective.

"When diet is wrong, medicine is of no use. When diet is correct, medicine is of no need".
Ayurvedic proverb

Migraine – A Case Study

Migraines can be incapacitating and arise from a variety of causes. The following is an account of how I worked with a client over a period of years to help manage her migraines. For reasons of confidentiality I refer to her as Laura.

I first met Laura in June 2010. She was referred to me through a project I was working with at the time for help with anxiety. She had a demanding job in the mental health sector with a lot of responsibility and very little support.

She had a history of depression, which was not present at the time we started working together, but she had developed acute anxiety. The greatest and most significant health problem she felt was recurrent migraines around her period, and the most recent episode was the day before our first meeting.
Her diet and lifestyle were fairly good, and she exercised quite regularly. Her periods were regular but she noticed hormonal fluctuations around them. Laura occasionally suffered from IBS symptoms and tended to be

constipated. She slept well but could struggle to get to sleep.

From the case history she gave me, I felt that the anxiety, constipation and possible hormonal imbalance were going to be the three main factors implicated in the persistent migraines. We agreed to begin with weekly treatments and to review this after 6 weeks.

Because I work on a bodily system by bodily system basis, it is very easy to tailor treatments to the specific needs of each client. I work in a holistic way, so I pay attention to each area of the body, but there is still plenty of room to make the treatments individual. For this particular client I generally emphasised the reflexes to do with stress and the nervous system, and also the hormones through the endocrine system. There is considerable overlap in these two areas. Reflexes of particular importance were the adrenal glands, which not are not only implicated in stress response, but tend to amplify any other issues.

Initially after treatment, Laura had a slight increase in anxiety which is not unusual, but found it calmed quickly. The low level constipation she had been suffering from was at least partly resolved the same day after a bowel movement. She found that in the week after the treatment she experienced an increased sense of wellbeing during the day. By the third treatment, Laura reported significantly less anxiety.

There was a 3 week break before the 4th treatment, and the client reported a low level feeling of stress. She had had a small migraine after the third treatment, but nothing around her period.

Laura had two more weekly treatments and then moved to having monthly top up treatments. Although she reported feelings of work related stress and feelings of tiredness, she did not experience a full migraine although she occasionally had the feeling she might get one. It wasn't until February 2011, eight months after she started having treatments that she had a migraine. After that she didn't experience anything more than slight symptoms until December 2011 when her marital problems reached a crisis point.

Laura continued to have monthly treatments during this time and her marriage did break up in May 2012 triggering a huge migraine. Over the next few months she had headaches and symptoms but no full migraines, so we worked hard at bringing her stress levels under control. She struggled with stress and anxiety for a while following the marital breakup but did not have another migraine until April 2013. Laura continued to struggle with work related stress and had another migraine 6 months later.

I continued working with Laura on a monthly basis until September 2015 when due to changes in circumstances we were no longer able to work together. After October 2013 she had no further migraines although she occasionally suffered with minor symptoms.

Over the course of the treatments we were able to restore some hormonal stability. It is my opinion that her migraines were extremely closely linked with her menstrual cycle, but that her stress and anxiety levels were the critical factor in whether or not she would have a full migraine. When her life was in a fairly good balance, her own self-care, coupled with regular Reflexology, meant that she didn't experience migraines on a monthly basis any more.

Part Three: Foot Healthcare

"Only a fool tests the depth of the water with both feet."
African proverb

What should you do if you have a pain in your foot?

I have a lot of clients calling me and saying "I have a pain in my foot. Can you help?" It is a hard question to answer.

There are an infinite variety of reasons why a person might have a pain somewhere in their foot, but they are not always obvious. Common culprits include: plantar fasciitis (damage to the band of tissue which runs under the foot) and poor fitting shoes. Often these problems can be resolved by the person themselves, but some may need additional treatment.

So if you have an unexplained pain in your foot here are some questions you can ask to determine whether you need further treatment. First of all look at the painful area. Can you see anything? Is it swollen or red? This would indicate inflammation, and would need further attention. Is there anything obvious there, like a corn or a blister? Is there a foreign object like a splinter or a fragment of glass? Is the skin broken? Is there blood or pus? Any of the above would indicate the need to seek further treatment from a GP or Foot Health Practitioner.

It is not always that simple. Sometimes there is nothing obvious on the foot to indicate what needs to be done. In these cases it is important to think about the history and character of the pain. Do your feet only hurt in the evening? Is it possible that they have been so cramped in the shoes you were wearing all day, that when they finally have room to breathe they start throbbing? Did they begin hurting after a particularly long walk, or when you started using a new pair of shoes? It is often amazing how easy it is to resolve these problems once you have taken the time to work out the root cause.

As a general rule of thumb, if you can see an obvious injury or problem on your foot, it would be a good idea to call a Foot Health Practitioner or a Podiatrist to ask their opinion. If the cause of the pain is not obvious it would be worth asking a Reflexologist.

Swimming Pools and Changing Rooms

You may have seen people wearing verruca socks while at the pool. You may have picked up athlete's foot a few times while changing at the gym. So what do we do about this?

The most important thing to remember is that, despite the best efforts of the staff to keep changing rooms and poolside clean, both the verruca virus and the athlete's foot fungus are rife.

As we will discuss later, the verruca is a virus which cannot be killed, and as an adult you are only likely to get it if you are run down. So in this case, the best thing to do is to look after your general health, and follow the treatment I suggest on Page 81. There is no point in avoiding pools or changing rooms as the virus is already there, and verruca socks have limited value.

There is more you can do to stop yourself picking up athlete's foot. There are many anti-fungal dusting powders you can buy, which you can use after you have showered and dried your feet thoroughly. One popular high street shop which sells bath and body products, has a powdered deodorant which I suspect would work very well, as it contains tea tree oil and thyme. I would also recommend using a good foot cream with peppermintt and tea tree oil.

The most important thing to remember is that you can't avoid coming into contact with verrucae and athlete's foot, and I would certainly not advise avoiding health centres. You can minimise your risk of catching and/or spreading them, so that should be the main aim.

Lotus Tips:

To minimize exposure to infection

- **Dry feet thoroughly**

- **Consider using an anti-fungal powder**

Runner's Foot Problems

It should be obvious to any serious runner that they need to look after their feet. After all, unlike other injuries, an injury to your foot can finish your season. The foot absorbs so much impact on landing, and stretches so much on take-off, that is surprising injuries don't happen more often.

For the purposes of this chapter I am going to categorise injuries as internal and external. Both can be helped, and often prevented, and that is what we are going to cover here.
By internal injuries I mean injuries which are beneath the surface of the skin. The principle ones are plantar fasciitis and Achilles tendonitis.

External injuries are less serious but still painful and debilitating. They include: calluses, black toenails and blisters.

What can we do about these problems? Well, the first thing to make sure of is that your running shoes are supportive and fit well. They should be measured properly in a specialist shop which will give the best recommendation based on your measurements.

One of the most common "internal" injuries experienced by runners, is plantar fasciitis. The most common causes are neglecting to stretch calf muscles properly, or overtraining, particularly hill work. The plantar fascia is a thick band of muscle running underneath the foot from the toes to the heel. It can tear due to overwork which will lead to painful inflammation, and will be very slow to heal.
At this point Reflexology would be recommended, to help reduce the inflammation and speed the healing process. Similarly Achilles tendonitis, which also arises from inflammation due to overwork, would benefit from Reflexology to speed the healing process.

"External" injuries are where the services of a Foot Health Practitioner would be most useful. A build-up of hard skin is an indication that your running shoes don't fit as well as they should. This can be because they didn't fit well in the first place, or because due to age and wear and tear they have lost some tension and support. The build-up of hard skin can be removed in minutes by a skilled practitioner.

Toenails can be injured by shoes that are too tight, or by shoes that are a little too big, allowing movement backwards and forwards in the shoe. This causes bruising, and can cause thickening of the nail. In either case the nail may fall off and re-grow. Thickened nails can be reduced in bulk by a Foot Health Practitioner, and this is advised, as they can become painful.

Blisters are also a sign that your running shoes do not fit well, but can also occur when people start training as the feet become used to the new demands made of them. The best treatment I have found is the application of pure aloe vera gel, which calms the pain quickly and helps the healing process.

Whether you are training for a big race, or just run for enjoyment, it is really important to properly care for your feet, and to address any small problems as they arise, so that they don't develop further.

Advice is like snow - the softer it falls, the longer it dwells upon, and the deeper it sinks into the mind.
Samuel Taylor Coleridge

High Heels

Let's be honest, they may look lovely but they are no good for you. I think most people know that wearing high heels is not good for the body, but I think many underestimate exactly how bad they are. And few realise the irreparable damage they are doing to their feet.

Let's start with the body; most people when they first start to wear high heels find them difficult to walk in. That is the first clue. They are hard to walk in because they change the whole posture of your body. Your feet are pushed into the shoe at an angle which, in order to keep your back straight you would have to lean forward. But no one wants to walk bent over, so we force ourselves to lean backwards, straining not only our spines, but all the muscles of our legs and back. When people wear high heels all the time the spine and muscles become habituated to this and we begin to think that everything is fine.

Some people even report that wearing flat shoes is painful, because they are so used to the way their body feels when wearing heels, that the normal has become abnormal.

The damage that is done to the feet is sometimes obvious immediately, but often not. In my practise it is usually fairly easy to tell that someone wears high heels a lot, because they usually have a large callus on the sole of their foot, around the metatarsal heads on the ball of the foot. This is often painful and a great relief to the client when removed. The feet build up this callus as a protection from the trauma of forcing the full weight of the body on to the toes and soles of the feet, instead of being spread over the whole foot.

Less obvious is the damage that is done to the toes. If your high heels have a pointed toe then it is likely you will develop corns on some of your toes. Our feet are quite round at the toe end, so forcing them into something narrow and pointed is likely to cause trouble. Some women develop hard corns on the side of the little toe, or on the tops of the toes. These are very painful and though they can be removed, they will keep returning if you force them into the same shoes that caused the problem, or indeed into any shoes that are too tight. Some people also develop soft corns in between the toes, which are caused by exactly the same pressure, and are also very painful.

There is also a type of damage done to the feet by high heels which does not become apparent until we are older. When forcing the toes into narrow pointed shoes and then forcing the toes and the soles to bear the whole weight of the body, we force the nails to rub against the shoe. This is a type of trauma, and the nail responds by building up extra layers, causing the nails to become thicker, and in some cases an awful lot.

Because it happens over time, and it doesn't tend to become apparent until later in life, people assume that it is because they are getting old, but this is not the case. Unless caused by some trauma, such as dropping a very heavy object onto a toe, thickened toenails are almost always caused by the repeated trauma of forcing the toes into shoes which are too narrow.

It is not up to me to dictate to people the kind of shoes they should choose. However, I really believe that people should make informed choices. The information I have given above, is based on my own experience, and the experience of practitioners who have been working in this field for a long time. If people choose to wear high-heels then they should know of the possible problems they are setting up for when they are older. My advice would be to severely limit wearing high heels to special occasions only.

*"Never bend your head. Always hold it high. Look the world straight in the face."
Helen Keller*

Natural treatment for a verruca

Verrucae are one of the more common things I have enquiries about in my Foot Health practice, which is hardly surprising as they are one of the most common problems people encounter on their feet.

Here's the thing; in my opinion, no one should ever have to pay money for someone to treat a verruca. THEY DO NOT NEED TO BE TREATED. I have met countless people who have made repeated visits to different practitioners to have their verrucae treated, often for quite a lot of money. It is not necessary. I much prefer to advise people over the phone, let them try a natural treatment for verruca, and only see people in the clinic if the verruca has become painful.

Verrucae are a virus, much like a common cold. Once you have caught a verruca, most commonly during childhood, the virus will continue to live in your system until you die. You cannot kill a verruca, so there is little point going to great lengths in order to do so.

There are, however things you can do to encourage them to go away.

Firstly, it is important to remember that if you are getting verrucae as an adult, it is a sign that your immune system is weak and you may be run down. So eat healthily, drink plenty of water, and make sure you are getting plenty of rest. The best natural treatment for verruca is to make your body so healthy the virus cannot thrive in it.

One of the best home treatments for verrucae is tea tree oil. If you paint some tea tree on any and all verrucae on your feet, morning and evening, it does seem to discourage them from hanging around too much. You have to be absolutely fanatical about this, painting them twice a day until all signs of verrucae are gone. This is what I advise my clients to do, and it seems to work very well. Most people who try this find that it works with two or three months.

Occasionally you might have a verruca which is so large, and so inconveniently placed on the sole of the foot that it becomes really painful to walk on. In these cases, clients can come and see me in the clinic, where I will file away any hard skin that has built up around the offender, and then carefully reduce some of the bulk of the verruca itself. It is not very common to have a verruca this problematic, and nine times out of ten, I would say it is completely possible to treat verrucae at home, following the treatment I have outlined above.

Lotus Tips

- **Look at your general health**
- **Eat plenty of nutrient rich food**
- **Consider taking a supplement**
- **Paint all verrucae with tea tree oil twice a day**

"Be sure you put your feet in the right place, then stand firm. "
Abraham Lincoln

Hard Skin and Callus

Hard skin is probably one of the most common problems people suffer with on their feet, but in some ways it is not a problem but a solution. Hard skin forms on the feet in response to friction, often caused by our footwear. This triggers the process of abnormal keratinisation where the body generates extra layers of skin in areas which it believes need more protection. In this way hard skin on the feet serves a protective function, and indicates where the feet are coming under the greatest stress.

Wearing pointed shoes can cause patches of hard skin and callus on the side of the big toe. High heels cause large patches of callus on the sole of the feet. Flip flops tend to generate hard rough skin on the heel in the summer months.

While it serves a very useful function, hard thick calluses can be extremely painful, and also unsightly. As I have discussed before the ideal way to treat this is prevention, by looking at your footwear and making sure your shoes fit well.

Using cream on the feet will also do a lot of good. Using a general moisturising cream two or three times a day, will help limit dryness and cracking, especially around the heels. In the summer, if you wear flip flops or sandals that move, it is important to take care that fissures do not develop in the heel. These can not only be very sore, but are also extremely difficult to treat.

Many people use files and gadgets like mini cheese graters to remove excess hard skin. I would really recommend thinking twice about using such equipment. People tend to go too far when using these gadgets, and you can end up cutting your feet to ribbons. The chances are, that you haven't sterilised the device before using it, so if you do cut yourself you will be introducing bacteria into the area, and you could end up with a nasty infection.

Instead of using these types of home care gadgets, consider setting up a daily foot care routine, as you would for your face. In the bath or shower, use a pumice stone, or a gentle exfoliating scrub (without microbeads), and then after drying the skin thoroughly use a nice moisturiser. If you find it hard to remember to use a cream on your feet, put the pot next to where you would sit and have a cup of tea in the evening. That way you are guaranteed a reminder, just at the time when you are sitting down for 5 minutes.

Setting up this kind of daily routine will be a huge benefit if you like to wear flip flops in the summer. Flip flops are actually great for the feet (except if you are diabetic. See the section on diabetic feet P97), but the heels do pay the price of all that extra rubbing.

"Beauty's only skin deep, but ugly goes right through to the bone."
Dorothy Parker

Home-made Foot Scrub Recipe

Here is a very simple scrub recipe that you can make at home and use regularly to help slow the damage to your heels from wearing flip-flops. You can vary it by using different oils and essential oils to suit your tastes. I default to a minty scent because I like the freshness.

It is good to make a home-made scrub, because it reduces packaging waste, and contains no microbeads which are devastating to the marine life of our oceans.

1 cup sea salt or Epsom salt
½ cup coconut oil
6 drops essential oil

Make by mixing all the ingredients and storing in an airtight container.
This recipe makes loads so you can use it as a whole body scrub or reduce the quantity.

"It's not selfish to love yourself, take care of yourself, and to make your happiness a priority. It's necessary."
Mandy Hale

How to deal with corns

Corns are very much a "shoe shape" issue, in that the vast majority are caused by ill-fitting shoes. Although corns are often associated with women, I expect to see more and more men in my clinic with corns, as the population ages, and the trend for very narrow shoes continues.

Corns can be divided into three types: hard corns, soft corns and seed corns.

Hard corns are found on bony prominences, especially the toes. It is here that the result of wearing pointed shoes, high heels and court shoes for extended periods of time can most clearly be seen. They are usually very painful.

Soft corns are only found between the toes. They are literally soft because of their location, but they can still be extremely painful.

Seed corns occur on the bottom of the foot, and there is no clear reason why they appear. They can become large and painful, and do have a tendency to reoccur, unlike soft and hard corns, which usually go once the cause is removed.

When I am asked how to deal with corns I always advise that the best way is to remove the cause completely. That means looking at your footwear and replacing it with shoes that fit better and don't cause undue pressure in those areas. Unfortunately shoe manufacturers produce according to demand, and so most shoes are made with quite a narrow toe.

Time and time again in my clinic I hear people defend their shoes because they are comfortable, but this does not mean that the shoes are not causing the damage. Our feet become used to being cramped into shoes and we might not feel any obvious discomfort, but they can still be causing the problem.

When people ask how to deal with corns, often they are not prepared to take the action required and change their shoes.

If people are not prepared to change their footwear they often try over the counter remedies such as corn plasters and shoe inserts. Shoe inserts are in my view a mistake, and can either aggravate the problem or create another elsewhere. If the shoes are already too tight, introducing something else will only reduce space further. You could find yourself with another corn.

A lot of women like corn plasters, as they do seem to work, but they only work on a temporary basis, so if the cause is still present the corn will always come back. Personally I don't like them as they seem to leave the area quite raw.

I have a lot of regular clients with corns, who don't want to change their footwear and so come to me to have them removed. Filing down corns doesn't work, because the nucleus of the corn, the part which causes the pain, is like a small ball-bearing of hard skin which is being pushed into the foot by pressure. Filing only removes the top of the hard skin and doesn't get down to the nucleus. A skilled Foot Health Practitioner will remove all the hard skin and the nucleus of the corn, leaving the client pain free for many weeks. If the individual then changes their footwear the corn will not come back.

"As soon as healing takes place, go out and heal somebody else."
Maya Angelou

Fungal Nail Infections

Fungal nail infections or onychomycosis often show up as discoloration of the nails, or white soft patches on the nail. They are extremely common. This kind of infection can spread across the toes, and can result in the loss of the nail if allowed to progress unchecked.

There are many over the counter remedies, and prescribed medicines for fungal nails but the key with all of them persistence. If you discontinue treatment before the nail has grown through completely clear, it is highly likely that the fungus will re-infect. There are also systemic medicines available on prescription, but as they have very severe side effects, they should only be used as a last resort.

In my clinic I see a lot of people with some kind of fungal infection of the nail, and there are two remedies I like to recommend: the first is tea tree oil, which is well known for its antifungal properties, but the second is rather unusual. The podiatrist who trained me, Bernard Pink, told me that rubbing vaporub over the affected nails regularly, had really good results. I have been recommending this treatment to my clients now for some time, and I can say that every client who has used vaporub regularly on their affected nails, has seen a vast improvement, with the nails growing through clear, and with the area affected by the fungus reduced. The additional benefit of this is that vaporub is very inexpensive, and a pot will last for months, unlike any other treatment you can use.

Part of any Foot Health treatment is to reduce the thickness of any nails, and this is especially important with fungal nails. Reducing the thickness of the nails exposes the areas with the fungus, and allows whatever treatment people are using to be more easily absorbed, making it more effective.

The most important factor in the success of any treatment for fungal nails, is the persistence of the client. If they continue the treatment regularly, until the nails are growing through clear, then the infection will go.

Foot Care for Diabetics

Diabetes is a serious condition and it can be a shock to be diagnosed with it. How we look after our feet becomes even more important than usual for a person suffering from diabetes. Loss of sensation can occur in the feet due to the disease, and this combined with poor wound healing ability can lead to complications and infections. In the UK, most diabetics have access to a certain amount of free foot care, but here are some simple steps you should follow to help prevent problems building up.

• On a daily basis wash your feet carefully in WARM soapy water. To avoid risk of burning, it is safest to test the temperature with your elbow or a thermometer. If you have very dry skin, your GP can prescribe you an emulsion to use instead of soap. Dry your feet thoroughly, patting instead of rubbing.

• After washing every day, check your feet all over, looking for cracks, corns or blisters. If you have problems with your eyesight or mobility ask someone else to do this for you.

• If you find any problems deal with them

immediately. For some things, some antiseptic cream and a clean bandage will be enough. Make sure you see a GP or Foot Health Practitioner about any problems you find.

• It is important to wear clean socks or tights every day. Ensure there are no holes or large seams and that they are large enough. Wear soft shoes with plenty of room, with no features that could cause pressure or rubbing. Never go barefoot.

• Be careful to protect your feet from very hot or very cold conditions.

• When cutting toenails, do not cut down the sides of the nails, or poke anything down the sides like a file. If you have trouble cutting your own nails, it is important to see a Foot Health Practitioner who is trained professionally to do this for you.

• If you have any concerns about the condition of your feet or discover any problems you should see a Foot Health Practitioner or a GP as soon as possible.

Final Word

Thank you for reading this book. I hope you found it useful and that it has perhaps in a small way inspired you.

If you have been left with questions that is no bad thing. "A Single Step" was never intended to be an exhaustive and definitive text, but rather a gentle introduction.

My greatest hope is that you are armed with more knowledge than you began the book with, and that it will help you make more informed decisions.

If you are interested in learning more about any of the topics in this book, please feel free to connect with me on various social media platforms, the links for which are below:

Twitter: @LotusReflexolog
@ASingleStepBook

Facebook:
https://www.facebook.com/LotusReflexology/
https://www.facebook.com/ASingleStepTheBook

Website: www.lotusreflexology.co.uk

About the Author

Kate McEwan is a Reflexologist and Foot Health Practitioner based in Bristol.

Her passion for supporting people with a variety of health problems led her to work in the complementary healthcare industry. Since qualifying as a Member of the Association of Reflexologists in 2003, and as a Foot Health Practitioner in 2014, she has worked within organisations and privately.

Her extensive clinical experience with all kinds of foot and health problems inspired her to write this book, to help broaden understanding of complementary treatments.

Kate currently lives in Bristol and can be found in her spiritual home of the Liberty stadium in Swansea most weekends.

Printed in Great Britain
by Amazon